7 Days to a Trimmer Belly

Get Rid of Your Pounds, Repair Your Digestive System, and Experience a Lighter, Younger You.

Joseph J. Davidson

Table of Content

Introduction

Day 1

Detox Your Body and Boost Your Immune System

Day 2

Restore Your Gut Flora and Support Your Digestion and Nutrient Absorption

Day 3

Add Fiber and Protein to Your Diet and Increase Your Satiety, Regulate Your Blood Sugar, and Prevent Cravings and Overeating

Day 4

Incorporate Healthy Fats into Your Diet Nourish Your Cells, Hormones, and Brain, and Promote Fat Burning and Appetite Control.

Day 5

Reduce Stress and Inflammation in the Body and the Mind, and Improve Mood and Sleep Quality

Day 6

Add Super foods and Antioxidants to Your Diet Enhance Your Healing Process and Protect Your Body from Free Radicals and Oxidative Damage

Day 7

Celebrate Your Achievements and Plan for the Future

Introduction

Are you tired of feeling bloated, heavy, and sluggish? Do you want to get rid of your persistent belly fat, improve your digestion, and enjoy a lighter, younger you?

In this book, you will discover how to attain a trimmer belly, better digestion, and increased health in just 7 days. You will understand the mysteries of the gut, the second brain of the body, and how it impacts your weight, your mood, your immunity, and your overall well-being. You will also study the causes and effects of belly obesity, digestive difficulties, and inflammation, and how they are linked to numerous chronic diseases such as diabetes, heart disease, cancer, and Alzheimer's.

You will discover how to heal your gut and lose weight with a holistic strategy that involves nutrition, exercise, stress management, and supplements. You will follow a simple and efficient 7-day strategy that will help you detoxify your body, repair your gut flora, raise your metabolism, reduce your appetite, and burn your fat. You will also enjoy delicious and healthy dishes that will fuel your cells, hormones, and brain, and protect your body from free radicals and oxidative damage.

By the end of this book, you will feel lighter, leaner, and healthier. You will have greater energy, improved mood, and clearer skin. You will also have a stronger immune system, a lower chance of disease, and a longer lifetime. You will be amazed by the transformation that you may achieve in just 7 days!

So, what are you waiting for? Grab your copy of this book today and start your journey to a trimmer belly, a happy stomach, and a healthier you!

Day 1

Detox Your Body and Boost Your Immune System

Welcome to Day 1 of your 7-day journey to a trimmer belly, a happy gut, and a healthier you! Today, you will start with a light detox to clear your body of toxins, parasites, and yeasts that may be hurting your gut and causing bloating, gas, and constipation. You will also learn how to employ natural therapies such as lemon water, apple cider vinegar, ginger, garlic, and turmeric to flush out the pollutants and improve your immune system.

Why Detox?

Detoxification is the process of removing toxic compounds from your body that may collect over time due to exposure to environmental contaminants, chemicals, narcotics, alcohol, and processed foods. These compounds can interfere with your body's regular activities and create numerous symptoms such as fatigue, headaches, skin problems, allergies, and weight gain. They can also damage your gut lining and upset your gut flora, which are crucial for digestion, immunity, and overall health.

By detoxing your body, you may enhance your gut health and reduce inflammation, which are important components for decreasing belly fat and preventing chronic diseases. You can also increase your metabolism, energy, mood, and cognitive performance, and avoid infections and illnesses.

How to Detox?

There are various ways to detox your body, but some of them might be severe and induce unpleasant side effects such as nausea, diarrhea, and dehydration. In this book, we will employ a mild and natural approach that will neither deprive you of nutrients nor cause stress to your body. Instead, we will employ simple and efficient remedies that will assist your body's own detoxification mechanisms and help you eliminate the toxins safely and gently.

Some of the natural therapies that we will apply are:

• **Lemon water:** Lemon water is a terrific way to start your day, as it helps to alkalize your body, hydrate your cells, and stimulate your liver and kidneys, which are the main organs responsible for detoxification. Lemon water also contains vitamin C, which is a potent antioxidant that helps protect your body from free radicals and enhance your immune system. To create lemon water, simply squeeze half a lemon into a glass of warm water and drink it first thing in the morning on an empty stomach.

• **Apple cider vinegar:** Apple cider vinegar is another wonderful detox agent, as it helps to balance your pH levels, aid your digestion, and manage your blood sugar. Apple cider vinegar also includes acetic acid, which can fight dangerous bacteria and fungi in your gut and prevent infections and candida overgrowth. To use apple cider vinegar, mix one to two tablespoons of it with a glass of water and drink it before each meal.

• **Ginger:** Ginger is a pungent and aromatic root that has various health benefits, such as anti-inflammatory, anti-nausea, and anti-microbial characteristics. Ginger can assist to relax your stomach, ease gas and bloating, and boost your digestion and circulation. Ginger can also aid in fighting off colds and flu and reduce discomfort and inflammation in your joints and muscles. To utilize ginger, you may either add fresh or dried ginger to your tea, smoothies, soups, or salads, or you can make a ginger shot by mixing a small piece of ginger with some water and lemon juice and taking it as a shot.

• **Garlic:** Garlic is a potent natural antibiotic that can eliminate harmful bacteria, viruses, and parasites in your gut and body. Garlic can also assist in lowering your blood pressure, cholesterol, and blood sugar, and avoid blood clots and strokes. Garlic can also improve your immune system and protect you from infections and disorders. To use garlic, you can either eat a little piece of raw garlic every morning, or you can chop or crush some garlic and add it to your recipes, sauces, or dressings.

• **Turmeric:** Turmeric is a yellow spice that has potent anti-inflammatory and antioxidant benefits. Turmeric can help to reduce inflammation in your gut and body and protect your cells from oxidative damage. Turmeric can also aid in boosting your liver function, brain function, and mood. To utilize turmeric, you can either add a pinch of turmeric powder to your tea, smoothies, soups, or curries, or you can take a turmeric supplement or pill.

These are some of the natural therapies that you can take to detox your body and enhance your immune system. However, you should also pay attention to what you eat and drink during the day, since some foods and beverages might aid or impede your detox process.

What to Eat and Drink?

On Day 1, you should focus on eating and drinking foods and beverages that are fresh, natural, and organic, and that can assist in cleansing your body and feeding your gut. You should also avoid meals and beverages that contain gluten, dairy, sugar, and processed substances, as these can promote inflammation, allergies, and digestive disorders.

Here is a sample menu for the day that you can follow or adapt according to your preferences and availability:

- **Breakfast:** A glass of lemon water, followed by a green smoothie made with spinach, kale, cucumber, celery, apple, banana, ginger, and water.
- **Snack:** A handful of raw almonds and a cup of green tea with a slice of lemon.
- **Lunch:** A huge salad made with mixed greens, tomatoes, carrots, avocado, olives, and sunflower seeds, seasoned with apple cider vinegar, olive oil, garlic, and turmeric.
- **Snack:** A bowl of fresh berries and a cup of chamomile tea with a teaspoon of honey.

- **Dinner:** A vegetable soup made with broccoli, cauliflower, onion, garlic, ginger, turmeric, vegetable broth, and coconut milk.
- **Snack:** A cup of warm almond milk with a dash of cinnamon and nutmeg.

You can add some lemon, cucumber, mint, or berries to your water to make it more refreshing and delectable.

What to Do?

On Day 1, you should also engage in some basic activities that might help to stimulate your blood circulation and lymphatic drainage, which are necessary for detoxification and immunity. You should also avoid severe or vigorous exercises that can bring stress or injury to your body.

- **Walking:** Walking is a low-impact and easy activity that can assist in enhancing your cardiovascular health, burn calories, and reduce stress. Walking can also aid in oxygenating your blood, stimulate your lymphatic system, and increase your mood and vitality. You can walk for at least 30 minutes a day, especially in the morning or evening, and in a natural or scenic area.

- **Stretching:** Stretching is a mild and relaxing exercise that can assist in loosening up your muscles, joints, and tendons, and avoid stiffness and pain. Stretching can also assist in improving your posture, flexibility, and range of motion, and relieve tension and pain. You can stretch for at least 10 minutes a day, preferably before and after your walk, and focus on your neck, shoulders, back, chest, arms, legs, and hips.

- **Yoga:** Yoga is a comprehensive and attentive activity that can assist in balancing your body, mind, and soul, and harmonize your energy and emotions. Yoga can also assist to strengthen your core, tone your muscles, and enhance your breathing and digestion. You can practice yoga for at least 20 minutes a day, preferably in the morning or evening, and in a peaceful and comfortable area. You can follow a yoga video or app, or try some fundamental yoga positions such as the child's pose, the cat-cow pose, the downward-facing dog pose, the cobra pose, and the tree pose.

These are some of the activities that you can do on Day 1 to support your detox process and improve your immune system. However, you should also listen to your body and adapt your intensity and length according to your level and condition. You should also rest and sleep well, as sleep is vital for your body's repair and renewal.

Congratulations! You have completed Day 1 of your 7-day journey to a trimmer belly, a happy stomach, and a healthier you! You have done the first step to cleanse your body and increase your immune system, and you should feel pleased with yourself. You may feel some moderate detox symptoms such as headache, fatigue, or nausea, but these should disappear shortly as your body adjusts and heals. You may also notice some changes in your weight, appearance, and mood, as your body sheds the excess water, waste, and toxins. Keep up the excellent work and get ready for Day 2, where you will learn how to rebuild your gut flora and help your digestion and nutrient absorption. See you tomorrow!

Day 2

Restore Your Gut Flora and Support Your Digestion and Nutrient Absorption

Welcome to Day 2 of your 7-day journey to a trimmer belly, a happy gut, and a healthier you! Today, you will discover how to restore the balance of healthy bacteria in your gut and help your digestion and nutrition absorption. You will also understand the distinction between probiotics and prebiotics, and how they work together to create a healthy microbiome. You will also discover what foods are rich in probiotics and prebiotics, and how to incorporate them into your everyday diet.

Why Gut Flora?

Gut flora, also known as gut microbiota or gut microbiome, is the term used to describe the billions of bacteria that live in your digestive tract. These microorganisms include bacteria, fungi, viruses, and archaea, and they play a key part in your health and well-being.

Some of the roles of your gut flora are:

- **Digestion:** Your gut flora helps to break down the food you eat and extract the nutrients you need. It also helps to create some vitamins, such as vitamin K and B12, and some enzymes, such as lactase and cellulase.

- **Immunity:** Your gut flora helps to protect you from hazardous germs and toxins that may enter your body through your mouth or nose. It also helps to control your immune system and avoid inflammation and autoimmune illnesses.

- **Metabolism:** Your gut flora helps to manage your metabolism and influence your weight, appetite, and blood sugar. It also helps to manufacture various hormones, such as serotonin and dopamine, and alter your mood and behavior.

- **Genetics:** Your gut flora is unique to you and influenced by your genes, environment, nutrition, and lifestyle. It also affects your gene expression and epigenetics, which are the mechanisms that control how your genes are switched on or off.

As you can see, your gut flora is crucial for your health and well-being, and you should take good care of it. However, your gut flora can also be disrupted or harmed by other circumstances, such as stress, illness, medicine, food, and aging. When this happens, you may have numerous symptoms, such as bloating, gas, constipation, diarrhea, indigestion, acid reflux, food intolerance, allergies, skin problems, mood changes, weariness, and weight gain. You may also raise your risk of developing chronic conditions, such as irritable bowel syndrome, inflammatory bowel disease, diabetes, obesity, cardiovascular disease, and cancer.

To avoid or correct these disorders, you need to restore the balance of healthy bacteria in your gut and assist your digestion and nutrition absorption. One of the greatest methods to do this is to ingest probiotics and prebiotics, which are the two types of foods that may nurture and restore your gut flora.

What are Probiotics and Prebiotics?

Probiotics and prebiotics are two types of meals that can help to improve your gut health and function. They are sometimes described as the "dynamic duo" or the "symbiotic" of the gut, as they work together to create a healthy microbiome. Here is the difference between them:

- **Probiotics:** Probiotics are live bacteria that can give health advantages to the host when taken in suitable doses. Probiotics can assist in replacing the healthy bacteria in your gut and restore the balance of your gut flora. They can also assist in boosting your digestion, immunity, metabolism, and mood. Some of the common sources of probiotics are fermented foods, such as yogurt, kefir, sauerkraut, kimchi, and kombucha. You can also take probiotic pills or capsules, but make sure to choose a high-quality and renowned brand that contains numerous strains and billions of colony-forming units (CFUs) of probiotics.

- **Prebiotics:** Prebiotics are non-digestible carbohydrates that can increase the growth and activity of the beneficial bacteria in your stomach. Prebiotics can aid in feeding and nourishing the probiotics and boost their effects. They can also assist in boosting your digestion, immunity, metabolism, and mood. Some of the common sources of prebiotics are fiber-rich foods, such as bananas, oats, apples, asparagus, and onions. You can also take prebiotic supplements or powders, but make sure to choose a natural and organic product that contains inulin, fructooligosaccharides (FOS), or galactooligosaccharides (GOS).

By ingesting probiotics and prebiotics, you can establish a healthy and diversified microbiome that can help you attain a trimmer tummy, a happy gut, and a healthier you.

How to Eat Probiotics and Prebiotics?

On Day 2, you should focus on eating and drinking foods and beverages that are rich in probiotics and prebiotics, and that can assist in restoring and maintaining your gut flora. You should also avoid foods and beverages that may disturb or damage your gut flora, such as alcohol, caffeine, and antibiotics.

Here is a sample menu for the day that you can follow or adapt according to your preferences and availability:

- **Breakfast:** A bowl of plain yogurt with some granola, sliced bananas, and honey, followed by a glass of kefir or kombucha.
- **Snack:** A handful of dried fruits and nuts, and a cup of ginger tea with a teaspoon of apple cider vinegar.
- **Lunch:** A sandwich made with whole wheat bread, turkey, cheese, lettuce, tomato, and avocado, topped with some sauerkraut or kimchi, and a side of carrot and celery sticks with some hummus.

- **Snack:** A sliced apple with some peanut butter, and a cup of green tea with a slice of lemon.

- **Dinner:** A chicken and vegetable stir-fry made with onion, garlic, ginger, turmeric, broccoli, cauliflower, carrot, and chicken, served with some brown rice or quinoa, and a dollop of yogurt or sour cream.

- **Snack:** A cup of warm milk with a touch of cinnamon and nutmeg, and a piece of dark chocolate.

You can add some lemon, cucumber, mint, or berries to your water to make it more refreshing and delectable.

What to Do?

On Day 2, you should also engage in some moderate workouts that can assist in burning calories and enhance your cardiovascular health, which are crucial for your weight loss and well-being. You should also avoid excessive or vigorous exercises that can create stress or injury to your body.

- **Cycling:** Cycling is a fun and easy exercise that can assist in enhancing your cardiovascular health, burn calories, and tone your legs and glutes. Cycling can also assist to relieve stress and boost your mood and energy. You can cycle for at least 30 minutes a day, especially in the morning or evening, and in a natural or scenic area. You can use your own bike or borrow one from a bike-sharing service.

- **Swimming:** Swimming is a low-impact and pleasant workout that can assist in enhancing your cardiovascular health, burning calories, and toning your complete body. Swimming can also assist to relieve stress and boost your mood and energy. You can swim for at least 20 minutes a day, preferably in the morning or evening, and in a pool or a natural body of water. You can use your own swimsuit or borrow one from a friend or a facility.

- **Dancing:** Dancing is a fun and social work out that can assist in enhancing your cardiovascular health, burn calories, and tone your muscles and joints. Dancing can also assist in relieving stress and boost your mood and vitality. You can dance for at least 20 minutes a day, especially in the afternoon or evening, and in a studio or a club. You can choose your own type of dancing, such as salsa, hip hop, or ballet, or follow a dance video or app.

These are some of the workouts that you can take on Day 2 to support your gut health and function and increase your weight reduction and well-being. However, you should also listen to your body and adapt your intensity and length according to your level and condition. You should also rest and sleep well, as sleep is vital for your body's repair and renewal.

Congratulations! You have completed Day 2 of your 7-day journey to a trimmer belly, a happier stomach, and a healthier you! You have learned how to restore the balance of beneficial bacteria in your gut and help your digestion and nutrition absorption, and you should feel pleased with yourself. You may notice some advantages in your digestion, immunity, metabolism, and mood, as your gut flora becomes more balanced and diverse. Keep up the excellent work and get ready for Day 3, where you will learn how to add fiber and protein to your diet and enhance your fullness, regulate your blood sugar, and prevent cravings and overeating. See you tomorrow!

Day 3

Add Fiber and Protein to Your Diet and Increase Your Satiety, Regulate Your Blood Sugar, and Prevent Cravings and Overeating

Welcome to Day 3 of your 7-day journey to a trimmer belly, a happy stomach, and a healthier you! Today, you will discover how to add fiber and protein to your diet and boost your fullness, manage your blood sugar, and reduce cravings and overeating. You will also learn the benefits of fiber and protein for digestion, metabolism, and weight loss, and how they can help reduce belly fat and inflammation. You will also discover what foods are high in fiber and protein, and how to balance them in each meal and snack.

Why Fiber and Protein?

Fiber and protein are two types of foods that can help you achieve a smaller tummy, a happy stomach, and a healthier you. They are sometimes referred to as the "power duo" or the "macronutrients" of the diet, as they offer energy and structure to your body. Here are some of the benefits of fiber and protein for your health and well-being:

- **Fiber:** Fiber is the indigestible portion of plant meals that can aid in enhancing your digestion and bowel motions. Fiber can also assist in boosting your satiety, as it slows down the digestion and absorption of meals, and makes you feel full longer. Fiber can also assist in managing your blood sugar, as it minimizes spikes and crashes that can contribute to cravings and overeating. Fiber can also assist in lowering your cholesterol, blood pressure, and inflammation, and avoid cardiovascular disease and diabetes. Some of the common sources of fiber are beans, lentils, nuts, seeds, and berries.

- **Protein:** Protein is the building block of your body that can aid in repairing and maintaining your muscles, bones, skin, hair, and nails. Protein can also assist in boosting your fullness, as it takes longer to digest and requires more energy to burn than carbohydrates or fats. Protein can also assist in regulating your blood sugar, as it stabilizes the insulin and glucagon hormones that control your glucose levels. Protein can also assist in enhancing your metabolism, as it increases your thermogenesis and muscle mass, which are the components that affect how many calories you burn at rest. Protein can also assist in reducing your belly fat and inflammation, as it stimulates the production of growth hormone and testosterone, which are the hormones that promote fat burning and muscle building. Some of the common sources of protein are eggs, fish, chicken, tofu, and quinoa.

By ingesting fiber and protein, you may construct a balanced and enjoyable diet that can help you attain a smaller tummy, a happy stomach, and a healthier you.

How to Eat Fiber and Protein?

On Day 3, you should focus on eating and drinking foods and beverages that are high in fiber and protein, and that can assist to enhance your digestion, metabolism, and weight reduction. You should also avoid meals and beverages that are low in fiber and protein, such as refined carbs, fried foods, and sweets, as these can promote inflammation, allergies, and digestive disorders.

Here is a sample menu for the day that you can follow or adapt according to your preferences and availability:

- **Breakfast:** A scrambled egg with some spinach, cheese, and salsa, served with a slice of whole wheat toast and a glass of orange juice.

- **Snack:** A protein bar and a cup of coffee with some milk and stevia.

- **Lunch:** A lentil and vegetable soup with some parsley and lemon juice, served with whole wheat pita bread and a green salad with some olive oil and vinegar.

- **Snack:** A handful of mixed nuts and dried fruits, and a cup of herbal tea with a spoonful of honey.

- **Dinner:** A grilled fish with some lemon and dill, served with some quinoa and roasted broccoli and carrots.

- **Snack:** A cup of Greek yogurt with some blueberries and oats, and a piece of dark chocolate. You can add some lemon, cucumber, mint, or berries to your water to make it more refreshing and delectable.

What to Do?

On Day 3, you should also engage in some strength training exercises that can help to build muscle and tone your body, which are crucial for your weight reduction and well-being. You should also avoid excessive or vigorous exercises that can create stress or injury to your body.

- **Squats:** Squats are a terrific exercise that can help to strengthen your legs, glutes, and core, and improve your posture and balance. Squats can also aid in burning calories and fat, and shape your lower body. You can practice squats for at least 15 repetitions, preferably in the morning or evening, and in a spacious and comfortable environment. You can use your own body weight or add some dumbbells or a barbell to boost the intensity and challenge.

- **Lunges:** Lunges are another wonderful workout that can assist in strengthening your legs, glutes, and core, and improve your posture and balance. Lunges can also help to burn calories and fat and shape your lower body. You can practice lunges for at least 15 repetitions per leg, preferably in the morning or evening, and in a big and comfortable environment. You can use your own body weight or add some dumbbells or a barbell to boost the intensity and challenge.

- **Push-ups:** Push-ups are a classic workout that can help to build your chest, shoulders, arms, and core, and enhance your upper body strength and endurance. Push-ups can also aid in burning calories and fat, and tone your upper body. You can do push-ups for at least 10 repetitions, preferably in the morning or evening, and in a spacious and comfortable environment. You can utilize your own body weight or add additional variants, such as incline, decline, or diamond push-ups, to improve the intensity and challenge.
- **Planks:** Planks are a simple and effective workout that can assist in strengthening your core, back, and hips, and improve your stability and

alignment. Planks can also assist in burning calories and fat, and flatten your abdomen. You can do planks for at least 30 seconds, especially in the morning or evening, and in a spacious and comfortable environment. You can use your own body weight or add various variants, such as side, reverse, or mountain climber planks, to improve the difficulty and challenge.

These are some of the workouts that you can do on Day 3 to support your fiber and protein intake and increase your weight reduction and well-being. However, you should also listen to your body and adapt your intensity and length according to your level and condition. You should also rest and sleep well, as sleep is vital for your body's repair and renewal.

Congratulations! You have completed Day 3 of your 7-day journey to a trimmer belly, a happier gut, and a healthier you! You have learned how to add fiber and protein to your diet and boost your fullness, manage your blood sugar, and prevent cravings and overeating, and you should feel pleased with yourself. You may see some benefits in your digestion, metabolism, and weight reduction, as your fiber and protein consumption become more balanced and adequate. Keep up the good work and get ready for Day 4, where you will discover how to include healthy fats into your diet fuel your cells, hormones, and brain, and improve fat-burning and hunger management. See you tomorrow!

Day 4

Incorporate Healthy Fats into Your Diet Nourish Your Cells, Hormones, and Brain, and Promote Fat Burning and Appetite Control.

Welcome to Day 4 of your 7-day journey to a trimmer belly, a happy gut, and a healthier you! Today, you will discover how to incorporate healthy fats into your diet fuel your cells, hormones, and brain, and improve fat-burning and hunger control. You will also understand the difference between healthy fats and bad fats, and how they affect the gut, the heart, and the waistline. You will also find out what foods are rich in healthy fats, and how to use them in moderation and combination with other macronutrients.

Why Fats?

Fats are one of the three macronutrients that provide energy and structure to your body, along with carbohydrates and proteins.

Fats are also vital for your health and well-being, as they serve different tasks, such as:

- **Cell membrane:** Fats are the main component of your cell membrane, which is the outer layer that protects and regulates your cells. Fats serve to maintain the fluidity and integrity of your cell membrane and allow the movement of nutrients, oxygen, and messages in and out of your cells.

- **Hormone synthesis:** Fats are the precursor of numerous hormones, such as estrogen, testosterone, cortisol, and thyroid hormones, which are the chemical messengers that control your growth, development, metabolism, reproduction, and stress response. Fats help to manufacture and balance your hormones and avoid hormonal abnormalities and illnesses.

- **Brain function:** Fats are the principal source of fuel for your brain, which is the organ that governs your cognition, memory, emotion, and behavior. Fats offer energy and protection for your brain and enhance your neuronal communication and development. Fats also help to manufacture some neurotransmitters, such as serotonin and dopamine, which are the molecules that regulate your mood and motivation.

- **Fat-soluble vitamins:** Fats are the carrier of some vitamins, such as vitamins A, D, E, and K, which are the vitamins that are soluble in fat and not in water. Fats help to absorb and distribute these vitamins to your tissues and organs and prevent vitamin deficits and disorders.

- **Essential fatty acids:** Fats are the source of some fatty acids, such as omega-3 and omega-6, which are the fatty acids that your body cannot generate and must acquire from your diet. Fats serve to give these vital fatty acids, which are important for your inflammation, immunity, and cardiovascular health.

As you can see, fats are necessary for your health and well-being, and you should not avoid or fear them. However, you should also realize that not all fats are created equal, and some fats are better than others for your gut, your heart, and your waistline.

What are Healthy Fats and Unhealthy Fats?

Fats can be categorized into numerous categories, based on their chemical structure and physical qualities. Some of the common forms of fats are:

- **Saturated fats:** Saturated fats are fats that have no double bonds between their carbon atoms, and are solid at room temperature. Saturated fats are generally found in animal products, such as meat, dairy, and eggs, and some plant items, such as coconut oil and palm oil. Saturated fats can raise your LDL (bad) cholesterol lower your HDL (good) cholesterol, and increase your risk of heart disease and stroke. You should limit your intake of saturated fats to fewer than 10% of your total calories per day, according to the World Health Organization (WHO).

- **Trans fats:** Trans fats are the fats that have been artificially changed by adding hydrogen atoms to their unsaturated bonds, and are solid or semi-solid at room temperature. Trans fats are typically present in processed foods, such as margarine, shortening, baked goods, fried foods, and snacks, and some animal products, such as dairy and meat. Trans fats can raise your LDL (bad) cholesterol lower your HDL (good) cholesterol, and increase your risk of heart disease, stroke, and diabetes. You should limit or minimize your intake of trans fats as much as possible, as they have no health benefits and only detrimental effects, according to the WHO.

- **Monounsaturated fats:** Monounsaturated fats are fats that have one double bond between their carbon atoms, and are liquid at normal temperature. Monounsaturated fats are generally present in plant items, such as olive oil, avocado, nuts, and seeds, and some animal products, such as fish and fowl. Monounsaturated fats can lower your LDL (bad) cholesterol boost your HDL (good) cholesterol, and minimize your risk of heart disease and stroke. You should incorporate some monounsaturated fats in your diet, as they have various health benefits and can enhance your gut, your heart, and your waistline.

- **Polyunsaturated fats:** Polyunsaturated fats are fats that contain more than one double bond between their carbon atoms, and are liquid at room temperature. Polyunsaturated fats are largely present in plant goods, such as sunflower oil, corn oil, soybean oil, and flaxseed oil, and some animal items, such as fish and shellfish. Polyunsaturated fats can lower your LDL (bad) cholesterol boost your HDL (good) cholesterol, and minimize your risk of heart disease and stroke. You should include some polyunsaturated fats in your diet, as they have various health benefits and can enhance your gut, your heart, and your waistline.

Among the polyunsaturated fats, two types of essential fatty acids are extremely necessary for your health and well-being, and they are:

- **Omega-3 fatty acids:** Omega-3 fatty acids are the fats that contain their first double bond at the third carbon atom from the end of the chain, and are liquid at room temperature. Omega-3 fatty acids are largely found in fish and seafood, such as salmon, tuna, sardines, and mackerel, and some plant items, such as flaxseed, chia seed, and walnuts. Omega-3 fatty acids can lessen your inflammation, increase your immunity, and protect your brain and heart. You should include some omega-3 fatty acids in your diet, as they have various health benefits and can enhance your gut, your heart, and your waistline.

- **Omega-6 fatty acids:** Omega-6 fatty acids are the fats that contain their first double bond at the sixth carbon atom from the end of the chain, and are liquid at room temperature. Omega-6 fatty acids are largely present in plant goods, such as sunflower oil, corn oil, soybean oil, and sesame oil, and some animal items, such as poultry and eggs. Omega-6 fatty acids can lessen your inflammation, increase your immunity, and protect your skin and hair. You should incorporate some omega-6 fatty acids in your diet, as they offer various health benefits and can enhance your gut, your heart, and your waistline.

However, you should also be aware that the ratio of omega-3 to omega-6 fatty acids in your diet is significant, as they have opposite impacts on your inflammation and immunity. Ideally, you should have a balanced ratio of omega-3 to omega-6 fatty acids, such as 1:1 or 2:1, according to some experts. However, most people have a skewed ratio of omega-3 to omega-6 fatty acids, such as 1:10 or 1:20, due to the use of processed foods and vegetable oils. This can create chronic inflammation and increase your risk of several diseases, including obesity, diabetes, and cancer. You should aim to lower your intake of omega-6 fatty acids and increase your intake of omega-3 fatty acids, to establish a balanced and healthy ratio.

By consuming healthy fats and avoiding bad fats, you may develop a balanced and nutritious diet that will help you attain a trimmer belly, a happy gut, and a healthier you.

How to Eat Healthy Fats?

On Day 4, you should focus on eating and drinking foods and beverages that are rich in healthy fats, including monounsaturated fats, polyunsaturated fats, and omega-3 fatty acids, and that can help to replenish your cells, hormones, and brain, and improve fat burning and hunger management. You should also avoid foods and beverages that are heavy in harmful fats, such as saturated fats, trans fats, and omega-6 fatty acids, as these can promote inflammation, allergies, and digestive disorders.

Here is a sample menu for the day that you can follow or adapt according to your preferences and availability:

- **Breakfast:** A smoothie made with avocado, spinach, almond milk, vanilla protein powder, and honey, followed by a boiled egg and a slice of whole wheat toast with some butter.

- **Snack:** A handful of walnuts and a cup of coffee with some coconut oil and stevia.

- **Lunch:** A salad made with mixed greens, cherry tomatoes, cucumber, olives, feta cheese, and salmon, seasoned with olive oil, lemon juice, garlic, and oregano.

- **Snack:** A celery stick with some peanut butter, and a cup of green tea with a slice of lemon.

- **Dinner:** A roasted chicken with some rosemary and thyme, along with some mashed cauliflower and roasted Brussels sprouts.

- **Snack:** A cup of Greek yogurt with some flaxseed and blueberries, and a piece of dark chocolate.

You can add some lemon, cucumber, mint, or berries to your water to make it more refreshing and delectable.

What to Do?

On Day 4, you should also engage in some high-intensity interval training (HIIT) activities that can aid in enhancing your metabolism and fat burning, which are crucial for your weight reduction and well-being. You should also avoid excessive or vigorous exercises that can create stress or injury to your body.

- **Sprinting:** Sprinting is a rapid and explosive activity that can assist in enhancing your cardiovascular health, burn calories, and fat, and tone your legs and glutes. Sprinting can also help to relieve stress and boost your mood and energy. You can run for at least 10 seconds, followed by 20 seconds of rest, and repeat for 10 rounds, preferably in the morning or evening, and in a big and safe place. You can utilize your own body weight or add additional resistance, such as a weighted vest or a sled, to increase the effort and challenge.

- **Jumping:** Jumping is a fun and dynamic workout that can assist in enhancing your cardiovascular health, burn calories and fat, and tone your complete body. Jumping can also assist in relieving stress and boost your mood and vitality. You can jump for at least 20 seconds, followed by 10 seconds of rest, and repeat for 10 rounds, preferably in the morning or evening, and in a big and safe place. You can utilize your own body weight or add additional variants, such as jumping jacks, jump squats, or jump lunges, to increase the resistance and challenge.

- **Burpees:** Burpees are a demanding and effective exercise that can assist in enhancing your cardiovascular health, burn calories and fat, and tone your complete body. Burpees can also assist to relieve stress and boost your mood and vitality. You can execute burpees for at least 15 seconds, followed by 15 seconds of rest, and repeat for 10 rounds, preferably in the morning or evening, and in a spacious and safe environment. You can utilize your own body weight or add some variants, such as push-up burpees, mountain climber burpees, or Spiderman burpees, to increase the difficulty and challenge.

These are some of the workouts that you can do on Day 4 to support your healthy fat consumption and increase your weight reduction and well-being. However, you should also listen to your body and adapt your intensity and length according to your level and condition. You should also rest and sleep well, as sleep is vital for your body's repair and renewal.

Congratulations! You have completed Day 4 of your 7-day journey to a trimmer belly, a happier gut, and a healthier you! You have learned how to incorporate good fats into your diet fuel your cells, hormones, and brain, and increase fat-burning and hunger management, and you should feel pleased with yourself. You may notice some gains in your energy, mood, and cognitive function, as your healthy fat consumption becomes more balanced and adequate. Keep up the good work and get ready for Day 5, where you will discover how to reduce stress and inflammation in the body and the mind and improve mood and sleep quality. See you tomorrow!

Day 5

Reduce Stress and Inflammation in the Body and the Mind, and Improve Mood and Sleep Quality

Welcome to Day 5 of your 7-day journey to a trimmer belly, a happy stomach, and a healthier you! Today, you will discover how to reduce stress and inflammation in the body and the mind and increase mood and sleep quality. You will also understand the connection between stress and inflammation, and how they might impact digestion, immunity, and weight reduction. You will also find out what ideas and techniques you may use to manage stress and inflammation, such as meditation, breathing, journaling, gratitude, and positive affirmations. You will also discover what foods might help lower stress and inflammation, such as dark chocolate, green tea, berries, and turmeric, and how to enjoy them as treats or supplements.

Why Stress and Inflammation?

Stress and inflammation are two interrelated phenomena that can affect your health and well-being, and your stomach, your heart, and your waistline. Stress is the body's response to any perceived or real threat or challenge, and it can be physical, mental, or emotional. Inflammation is the body's response to any damage or infection, and it can be acute or chronic. Here are some of the impacts of stress and inflammation on your body and mind:

- **Digestion:** Stress and inflammation can hinder your digestion and create different symptoms, such as bloating, gas, constipation, diarrhea, indigestion, acid reflux, and food intolerance. Stress can activate your sympathetic nervous system, which is the fight-or-flight response, and block your parasympathetic nervous system, which is the rest-and-digest response. This can reduce your blood supply and oxygen to your digestive organs, and slow down your digestive processes. Inflammation can damage your gut lining and upset your gut flora, which is vital for digestion, immunity, and overall health. This can lead to leaky gut syndrome, which is the condition where your gut becomes more porous and allows toxins, bacteria, and food particles to enter your circulation and trigger systemic inflammation and immunological reactions.

- **Immunity:** Stress and inflammation can damage your immunity and raise your risk of infections and disorders. Stress can depress your immune system and make you more sensitive to infections and poisons that may enter your body through your mouth or nose. Inflammation can overstimulate your immune system and cause it to attack your own tissues and organs, and develop autoimmune illnesses, such as rheumatoid arthritis, lupus, and celiac disease.

- **Metabolism:** Stress and inflammation can disrupt your metabolism and alter your weight, appetite, and blood sugar. Stress can boost your cortisol levels, which is the stress hormone that can increase your appetite, cravings, and fat storage, especially in your belly area. Inflammation can increase your insulin resistance, which is the situation when your cells become less receptive to insulin, which is the hormone that regulates your glucose levels. This can lead to high blood sugar, diabetes, and obesity.

- **Mood:** Stress and inflammation can disrupt your mood and alter your cognition, memory, emotion, and behavior. Stress can decrease your serotonin and dopamine levels, which are the neurotransmitters that regulate your mood and motivation. Inflammation can increase your cytokine levels, which are the inflammatory molecules that can pass your blood-brain barrier and alter your brain function and chemistry. This can lead to sadness, anxiety, and cognitive deterioration.

As you can see, stress and inflammation can have bad effects on your health and well-being, your gut, your heart, and your waistline. To avoid or reverse these disorders, you need to reduce stress and inflammation in your body and mind and enhance your mood and sleep quality. One of the greatest ways to achieve this is to employ some strategies and techniques that can help you manage stress and inflammation, such as meditation, breathing, journaling, gratitude, and positive affirmations.

What are Meditation, Breathing, Journaling, Gratitude, and Positive Affirmations?

Meditation, breathing, journaling, gratitude, and positive affirmations are some of the suggestions and strategies that can help you reduce stress and inflammation in your body and mind, and improve your mood and sleep quality. They are sometimes referred to as the "mindfulness practices" or the "self-care practices" of the body and mind, as they enable you to be more aware and compassionate of yourself and your environment.

Here are some of the benefits of these practices:

- **Meditation:** Meditation is the discipline of focusing your attention on a single object, such as your breath, a word, a sound, or a sensation, and observing your thoughts and feelings without judgment or reaction. Meditation can help you reduce stress and inflammation since it can lower your cortisol and cytokine levels, and boost your endorphin and oxytocin levels, which are the hormones that can make you feel calm, joyful, and connected. Meditation can also help you to enhance your mood and sleep quality, as it can increase your serotonin and melatonin levels, which are the hormones that can regulate your mood and sleep cycle. Meditation can also help you to improve your digestion, immunity, and metabolism since it can strengthen your parasympathetic nervous system, which is the rest-and-digest response. To practice meditation, you can sit or lie down in a comfortable and quiet spot, focus on your breath, a word, a sound, or a sensation, and let go of any distractions or judgments. You can meditate for at least 10 minutes a day, preferably in the morning or evening, and utilize a meditation app or video to guide you.

- **Breathing:** Breathing is the process of breathing and exhaling air through your nose or mouth, and it is necessary for your life and health. Breathing can help you to reduce stress and inflammation, as it can lower your blood pressure, heart rate, and muscular tension, and boost your blood oxygen and carbon dioxide levels, which can balance your pH levels and reduce acidity and inflammation. Breathing can also help you to improve your mood and sleep quality, as it can activate your vagus nerve, which is the nerve that connects your brain and your gut, and can modify your mood and sleep. Breathing can also aid you in improving your digestion, immunity, and metabolism, as it can strengthen your parasympathetic nervous system, which is the rest-and-digest response. To practice breathing, you can sit or lie down in a comfortable and quiet place, breathe deeply and slowly through your nose or mouth, and fill your lungs and abdomen with air. You can breathe for at least 5 minutes a day, especially in the morning or evening, and utilize a breathing app or video to guide you.

- **Journaling:** Journaling is the process of putting down your thoughts, feelings, and experiences on a paper or a digital device, and reflecting on them. Journaling can help you to reduce stress and inflammation, as it can enable you to express and release your feelings and cope with your challenges and problems. Journaling can also help you to enhance your mood and sleep quality, as it can help you to acquire insight and perspective and find meaning and purpose. Journaling can also help you to improve your digestion, immunity, and metabolism since it can allow you to discover and change your negative habits and behaviors. To practice journaling, you can write down anything that comes to your mind, such as your goals, dreams, anxieties, joys, or thankfulness, and reflect on them. You can journal for at least 10 minutes a day, preferably in the morning or evening, and use a journal app or notepad to record your entries.

- **Gratitude:** Gratitude is the habit of being thankful and appreciative of what you have and what you experience, and expressing it to yourself or others. Gratitude can help you to reduce stress and inflammation, as it can help you to change your emphasis from what you lack to what you have, and from what you can't control to what you can. Gratitude can also help you to improve your mood and sleep quality, as it can help you to foster positive emotions, such as happiness, joy, and love, and boost your social interactions and support. Gratitude can also help you enhance your digestion, immunity, and metabolism, as it can help you boost your self-esteem and self-care. To practice thankfulness, you can think of or write down three things that you are glad for each day, such as your health, your family, or your possibilities, and feel or express your thanks. You can practice appreciation for at least 5 minutes a day, preferably in the morning or evening, and use a gratitude app or journal to record your entries.

- **Positive affirmations:** Positive affirmations are the practice of repeating positive and uplifting statements to yourself or others, and believing in them. Positive affirmations can help you reduce stress and inflammation, as they can help you reprogram your subconscious mind and transform your negative ideas and thoughts. Positive affirmations can also help you to enhance your mood and sleep quality, as they can help you to raise your confidence, motivation, and optimism, and attain your goals and aspirations. Positive affirmations can also help you to improve your digestion, immunity, and metabolism, as they can enable you to strengthen your self-image and self-love. To practice positive affirmations, you might choose or make some phrases that resonate with you and your situation, such as "I am strong and capable", "I am worthy and deserving", or "I am healthy and happy", and repeat them to yourself or others. You can practice positive affirmations for at least 5 minutes a day, especially in the morning or evening, and utilize a positive affirmation app or audio to guide you.

These are some of the suggestions and techniques that you may use to reduce stress and inflammation in your body and mind and enhance your mood and sleep quality.

However, you should also realize that some foods might assist or hamper your stress and inflammation levels, and your mood and sleep quality.

What are Anti-Inflammatory Foods and Pro-Inflammatory Foods?

Anti-inflammatory meals and pro-inflammatory foods are two types of foods that can alter your stress and inflammation levels, and your mood and sleep quality. Anti-inflammatory foods are the foods that can help to reduce inflammation and promote healing in your body and mind. Pro-inflammatory foods are foods that can induce or increase inflammation and cause damage to your body and mind. Here are some of the common anti-inflammatory foods and pro-inflammatory foods:

- **Anti-inflammatory foods:** Anti-inflammatory foods are foods that are high in antioxidants, phytochemicals, and omega-3 fatty acids, which are substances that may neutralize free radicals, modulate inflammation, and protect your cells and tissues.

Some of the common anti-inflammatory foods are dark chocolate, green tea, berries, and turmeric. Dark chocolate is a delightful treat that can help to reduce stress and inflammation since it contains flavonoids, which are antioxidants that can increase your blood flow, lower your blood pressure, and enhance your mood and cognition. Green tea is a delicious beverage that can help to reduce stress and inflammation since it includes catechins, which are the antioxidants that can suppress the enzymes that make inflammatory chemicals, and enhance your immunity and metabolism. Berries are a delicious and juicy snack that can help to reduce stress and inflammation since they include anthocyanins, which are antioxidants that can reduce oxidative stress, lower your blood sugar, and improve your memory and learning. Turmeric is a yellow spice that can help to reduce stress and inflammation since it includes curcumin, which is the phytochemical that can block the pathways that produce inflammatory molecules, and enhance your digestion, immunity, and mood.

- **Pro-inflammatory foods:** Pro-inflammatory foods are foods that are heavy in sugar, salt, fat, and additives, which are substances that can raise oxidative stress, activate inflammation, and harm your cells and tissues. Some of the frequent pro-inflammatory foods are spicy, acidic, and caffeinated foods. Spicy meals are foods that contain capsaicin, which is a substance that can irritate your gut lining and produce inflammation and pain. Acidic foods are foods that have a low pH that can raise the acidity in your body and cause inflammation and acidosis. Caffeinated foods are foods that include caffeine, which is a stimulant that can boost your cortisol levels and induce stress and inflammation.

By consuming anti-inflammatory foods and avoiding pro-inflammatory foods, you may develop a balanced and healing diet that can help you attain a trimmer tummy, a happy gut, and a healthier you.

How to Eat Anti-Inflammatory Foods?

On Day 5, you should focus on eating and drinking foods and beverages that are rich in anti-inflammatory ingredients, such as antioxidants, phytochemicals, and omega-3 fatty acids, and that can help to reduce stress and inflammation in your body and mind and enhance your mood and sleep quality. You should also avoid foods and beverages that are high in pro-inflammatory ingredients, such as sugar, salt, fat, and additives, as they can cause or increase stress and inflammation in your body and mind, and damage your mood and sleep quality.

Here is a sample menu for the day that you can follow or adapt according to your preferences and availability:

- **Breakfast:** A bowl of oats with some almond milk, blueberries, and walnuts, followed by a cup of green tea with some honey and lemon.

- **Snack:** A piece of dark chocolate and a cup of chamomile tea with a spoonful of honey.

- **Lunch:** A chicken and vegetable curry made with onion, garlic, ginger, turmeric, cumin, coriander, coconut milk, chicken, and cauliflower, served with either brown rice or naan bread.

- **Snack:** A handful of mixed berries and a cup of ginger tea with a slice of lemon.

- **Dinner:** A salmon and vegetable salad composed of mixed greens, cherry tomatoes, cucumber, avocado, olives, feta cheese, and salmon, seasoned with olive oil, lemon juice, garlic, and oregano.

- **Snack:** A cup of warm milk with a touch of cinnamon and nutmeg, and a piece of dark chocolate.

You can add some lemon, cucumber, mint, or berries to your water to make it more refreshing and delectable.

What to Do?

On Day 5, you should also engage in some calming exercises that can assist in releasing stress and promote flexibility in your body and mind, which are crucial for your weight reduction and well-being. You should also avoid excessive or vigorous exercises that can create stress or injury to your body.

- **Tai chi:** Tai chi is a soft and graceful workout that can help to improve your balance, coordination, and posture, and reduce stress and inflammation. Tai chi can also assist in improving your mood and sleep quality since it can harmonize your energy and emotions, and encourage relaxation and peace. You can practice tai chi for at least 20 minutes a day, preferably in the morning or evening, and in a spacious and tranquil environment. You can utilize your own body weight or add additional accessories, such as a fan or a sword, to increase the resistance and challenge. You can follow a tai chi video or app, or join a tai chi class or group.

- **Pilates:** Pilates is a low-impact and effective workout that can help strengthen your core, tone your muscles, and improve your flexibility and alignment. Pilates can also help to reduce stress and inflammation, as it can improve your breathing and circulation, and lower your blood pressure and heart rate. Pilates can also assist in improving your mood and sleep quality since it can increase your endorphin and serotonin levels, and promote your self-esteem and self-confidence. You can do pilates for at least 20 minutes a day, preferably in the morning or evening, and in a spacious and comfortable environment. You can utilize your own body weight or add additional equipment, such as a mat, a ball, or a band, to increase the resistance and challenge. You can follow a Pilates video or app, or attend a Pilates class or studio.

- **Massage:** Massage is a peaceful and relaxing practice that can assist in easing pain and stiffness, and enhance your blood flow and lymphatic drainage. Massage can also help to reduce stress and inflammation, as it can lower your cortisol and cytokine levels, and boost your endorphin and oxytocin levels, which are the hormones that can make you feel relaxed, joyful, and connected. Massage can also assist in improving your mood and sleep quality, as it can increase your serotonin and melatonin levels, which are the hormones that can regulate your mood and sleep cycle. You can massage yourself or have someone massage you for at least 10 minutes a day, especially in the evening or before bed, and in a cozy and quiet environment. You can use your own hands or various instruments, such as a roller, a ball, or a stick, to impart pressure and movement to your muscles and joints. You can also use some oil, lotion, or cream, to lubricate and nourish your skin.

These are some of the activities that you can take on Day 5 to support your anti-inflammatory diet and increase your weight loss and well-being. However, you should also listen to your body and adapt your intensity and length according to your level and condition. You should also rest and sleep well, as sleep is vital for your body's repair and renewal.

Congratulations! You have completed Day 5 of your 7-day journey to a trimmer belly, a happier stomach, and a healthier you! You have learned how to minimize stress and inflammation in the body and the mind and enhance your mood and sleep quality, and you should feel pleased with yourself. You may see some improvements in your energy, mood, and cognitive performance, as your stress and inflammation levels become more balanced and lowered. Keep up the good work and get ready for Day 6, where you will learn how to cleanse your body and mind, and eliminate toxins and waste. See you tomorrow!

Day 6

Add Super foods and Antioxidants to Your Diet Enhance Your Healing Process and Protect Your Body from Free Radicals and Oxidative Damage

Welcome to Day 6 of your 7-day journey to a trimmer belly, a happy stomach, and a healthier you! Today, you will discover how to incorporate super foods and antioxidants to process and protect your body from free radicals and oxidative damage. You will also understand the benefits of super foods and antioxidants for the stomach, the skin, and overall health, and how they can help prevent and reverse aging and disease. You will also discover what foods are considered super foods and antioxidants, such as blueberries, spinach, kale, chia seeds, goji berries, and acai, and how to add them to smoothies, salads, and snacks.

Why super foods and Antioxidants?

Super foods and antioxidants are two types of nutrients that can accelerate your healing process and protect your body from free radicals and oxidative damage, which are the causes that can cause inflammation, aging, and illness. Super foods are foods that are rich in nutrients, such as vitamins, minerals, enzymes, and phytochemicals, which are substances that can support your body's processes and systems. Antioxidants are foods that are high in substances, such as flavonoids, carotenoids, and polyphenols, which are the compounds that may neutralize free radicals, which are unstable molecules that can damage your cells and tissues.

Here are some of the benefits of super foods and antioxidants for your body and mind:

- **Gut:** Super foods and antioxidants can boost your gut health and function, as they can give fiber, probiotics, and prebiotics, which are the compounds that can benefit your digestion, bowel movements, and gut flora. Super foods and antioxidants can help preserve your gut lining and prevent leaky gut syndrome, which is the condition where your gut becomes more porous and allows toxins, bacteria, and food particles to enter your circulation and trigger systemic inflammation and immunological reactions.

- **Skin:** Super foods and antioxidants can improve your skin health and beauty, as they can give collagen, elastin, and hyaluronic acid, which are the compounds that can improve your skin's structure, elasticity, and moisture. Super foods and antioxidants can also protect your skin from UV radiation, pollution, and stress, which are the causes that can cause skin damage, aging, and disease.

- **Overall health:** Super foods and antioxidants can improve your overall health and well-being, as they can provide various benefits, such as Boosting your immunity and preventing infections and diseases o Lowering your blood pressure, cholesterol, and blood sugar, and preventing cardiovascular disease and diabetes o Enhancing your brain function and memory and preventing cognitive decline and dementia o Improving your mood and energy and preventing depression and fatigue o Reducing your inflammation and pain and preventing arthritis and cancer

As you can see, super foods and antioxidants can have great effects on your health and well-being, and your gut, your skin, and your overall health. To gain these benefits, you need to include super foods and antioxidants in your diet and enjoy them as treats or supplements.

What are Super foods and Antioxidants?

Super foods and antioxidants are two types of foods that are rich in nutrients and compounds that can accelerate your healing process and protect your body from free radicals and oxidative damage. Some of the common super foods and antioxidants are:

- **Blueberries:** Blueberries are a tasty and juicy fruit that can help to reduce stress and inflammation since they include anthocyanins, which are the antioxidants that can reduce oxidative stress, lower your blood sugar, and improve your memory and learning. You can add blueberries to your smoothies, salads, or snacks, or eat them as they are.

- **Spinach:** Spinach is a leafy green food that can help to reduce stress and inflammation, as it contains lutein and zeaxanthin, which are the antioxidants that can protect your eyes and skin from UV radiation and pollution. Spinach also provides iron, folate, and vitamin K, which are the elements that can assist your blood, bones, and muscles. You may add spinach to your smoothies, salads, or soups, or sauté it with little garlic and olive oil.

- **Kale:** Kale is another leafy green vegetable that can assist in lowering stress and inflammation, as it includes glucosinolates, which are the phytochemicals that can modify your inflammation and detoxification pathways. Kale also contains vitamin C, vitamin A, and calcium, which are the elements that help strengthen your immune, skin, and bones. You may add kale to your smoothies, salads, or chips, or roast it with some salt and oil.

- **Chia seeds:** Chia seeds are tiny and crunchy seeds that can help to reduce stress and inflammation since they include omega-3 fatty acids, which are the vital fatty acids that can lower your inflammation, strengthen your immunity, and protect your brain and heart. Chia seeds also contain fiber, protein, and antioxidants, which are the chemicals that can enhance your digestion, satiety, and metabolism. You can add chia seeds to your smoothies, salads, or puddings, or soak them in water or milk.

- **Goji berries:** Goji berries are a sweet and chewy fruit that can help to reduce stress and inflammation since they include polysaccharides, which are the antioxidants that can enhance your immune, blood sugar, and mood. Goji berries also contain vitamin C, iron, and zinc, which are the nutrients that can help your skin, vitality, and wound healing. You can add goji berries to your smoothies, salads, or granola, or enjoy them as they are.

- **Acai:** Acai is a dark and pulpy berry that can help to reduce stress and inflammation, as it includes anthocyanins, which are the antioxidants that can protect your cells and tissues from free radical damage. Acai also contains fiber, protein, and omega-3 fatty acids, which are the elements that can aid your digestion, satiety, and metabolism. You may add acai to your smoothies, bowls, or sorbets, or have it as a juice.

These are some of the super foods and antioxidants that you can add to your diet and enjoy as treats or supplements. However, you should also realize that some meals might create oxidative stress and inflammation in your body and mind, and damage your mood and sleep quality.

What are Oxidative Stress and Inflammation Foods?

Oxidative stress and inflammation foods are foods that are high in chemicals that can boost free radical generation, stimulate inflammation, and harm your cells and tissues. Some of the common oxidative stress and inflammatory foods are:

- **Processed meats:** Processed meats are the meats that have been cured, smoked, salted, or preserved, such as bacon, ham, sausage, and salami. Processed meats can induce oxidative stress and inflammation since they include nitrites, which are the preservatives that can react with your stomach acid and generate nitrosamines, which are the carcinogens that can harm your DNA and cells. Processed meats also include heme iron, which is the form of iron that can promote free radical generation and oxidative stress. Processed meats also contain saturated fat, which is the sort of fat that can increase your LDL (bad) cholesterol and inflammation.

- **Fried foods:** Fried foods are foods that have been cooked in hot oil, such as French fries, chicken nuggets, and doughnuts. Fried meals can promote oxidative stress and inflammation, as they contain trans fats, which are the lipids that have been artificially changed by adding hydrogen atoms to their unsaturated bonds, and are solid or semi-solid at room temperature. Trans fats can raise your LDL (bad) cholesterol lower your HDL (good) cholesterol, and increase your risk of heart disease, stroke, and diabetes. Fried meals also contain acrylamide, which is the chemical that can occur when starchy foods are fried at high temperatures and can cause cancer and nerve damage.

- **Artificial sweeteners:** Artificial sweeteners are the compounds that are used to sweeten meals and beverages without adding calories, such as aspartame, sucralose, and saccharin. Artificial sweeteners can induce oxidative stress and inflammation since they can affect your gut flora and increase your blood sugar and insulin levels, which can lead to metabolic syndrome and diabetes. Artificial sweeteners can also alter your brain function and mood, as they can interfere with your serotonin and dopamine levels, which are the neurotransmitters that regulate your mood and motivation.

By eliminating oxidative stress and inflammation in meals and consuming super foods and antioxidant foods, you may develop a balanced and healing diet that can help you attain a trimmer belly, a happy gut, and a healthier you.

How to Avoid Oxidative Stress and Inflammation Foods?

On Day 6, you should avoid eating and drinking foods and beverages that are high in compounds that might induce oxidative stress and inflammation in your body and mind, and impact your mood and sleep quality, such as processed meats, fried foods, and artificial sweeteners. You should also limit your intake of other foods and beverages that can promote or increase oxidative stress and inflammation, such as spicy, acidic, and caffeinated foods.

Here is a sample menu for the day that you can follow or adapt according to your preferences and availability:

- **Breakfast:** A smoothie bowl made with acai, banana, almond milk, and chia seeds, topped with some granola, goji berries, and coconut flakes, followed by a cup of green tea with some honey and lemon.

- **Snack:** A handful of almonds and a cup of blueberry juice with a spoonful of honey.

- **Lunch:** A kale and quinoa salad made with kale, quinoa, cherry tomatoes, cucumber, avocado, and walnuts, drizzled with olive oil, lemon juice, garlic, and turmeric.

- **Snack:** A piece of dark chocolate and a cup of chamomile tea with a slice of lemon.
- **Dinner:** A spinach and salmon wrap made with spinach, salmon, cream cheese, and whole wheat tortilla, served with some carrot and celery sticks with some hummus.
- **Snack:** A cup of warm milk with a touch of cinnamon and nutmeg, and a piece of dark chocolate. You can add some lemon, cucumber, mint, or berries to your water to make it more refreshing and delectable.

What to Do?

On Day 6, you should also engage in some pleasant workouts that can assist you in enjoying nature and socializing with others, which are crucial for your weight loss and well-being. You should also avoid excessive or vigorous exercises that can create stress or injury to your body.

- **Hiking:** Hiking is a terrific activity that can assist you to visit new locations, breathe fresh air, and view stunning landscapes. Hiking can also enable you to burn calories and fat and tone your legs and glutes. Hiking can also help you to reduce stress and inflammation since it can improve your endorphin and serotonin levels, and enhance your mood and cognition. You can hike for at least 30 minutes a day, preferably in the morning or evening, and in a safe and scenic region. You can utilize your own body weight or add some equipment, such as a backpack, a pole, or a water bottle, to increase the resistance and difficulty. You can follow a hiking map or app, or join a hiking club or group.

- **Skating:** Skating is a pleasant and dynamic activity that can assist you to glide on ice or wheels, and feel the pleasure and excitement. Skating can also enable you to burn calories and fat and tone your complete body. Skating can also help you to reduce stress and inflammation since it can improve your endorphin and dopamine levels, and enhance your mood and vitality. You can skate for at least 20 minutes a day, especially in the afternoon or evening, and in a big and smooth location. You can utilize your own body weight or add additional equipment, such as a helmet, a pair of skates, or protective gear, to boost the safety and challenge. You can follow a skating video or app, or join a skating class or club.

- **Playing sports:** Playing sports is a social and competitive exercise that can allow you to engage with others, have fun, and challenge yourself. Playing sports can also enable you to burn calories and fat, and tone your muscles and joints. Playing sports can also help you to reduce stress and inflammation since it can improve your endorphin and oxytocin levels, and enhance your mood and relationships. You can do sports for at least 30 minutes a day, preferably in the afternoon or evening, and in a good and safe environment. You can utilize your own body weight or add additional equipment, such as a ball, a racket, or a net, to increase the resistance and challenge. You can follow a sports video or app, or join a sports team or club.

These are some of the workouts that you can take on Day 6 to support your super foods and antioxidants diet and increase your weight loss and well-being. However, you should also listen to your body and adapt your intensity and length according to your level and condition. You should also rest and sleep well, as sleep is vital for your body's repair and renewal.

Congratulations! You have completed Day 6 of your 7-day journey to a trimmer belly, a happier gut, and a healthier you! You have learned how to add super foods and antioxidants to your diet accelerate your healing process and protect your body from free radicals and oxidative damage, and you should feel pleased with yourself. You may notice some changes in your skin, hair, and nails, as your super food and antioxidant intake become more numerous and varied. Keep up the good work and get ready for Day 7, where you will learn how to celebrate your victories and maintain your outcomes. See you tomorrow!

Day 7

Celebrate Your Achievements and Plan for the Future

Welcome to Day 7 of your 7-day journey to a trimmer belly, a happy stomach, and a healthier you! Today, you will celebrate your achievements and plan for the future. You will assess the accomplishments and results that you have made in the past week, and congratulate yourself for taking action and making great changes in your life. You will also find out what strategies and advice you can use to maintain and enhance your gut health and weight reduction in the long run, such as keeping a food diary, setting reasonable goals, tracking your measurements, and rewarding yourself. You will also enjoy a sample menu for the day that contains your favorite foods from the previous days, and allow yourself some indulgences in moderation. You will also do some restorative exercises such as stretching, foam rolling, and meditation to heal and refresh.

Why Celebrate and Plan?

Celebrating and planning are two crucial activities that can enable you to sustain and optimize your gut health and weight loss, and your general health and well-being. Celebrating can assist you in acknowledging and appreciating your efforts and achievements, and enhance your confidence, motivation, and happiness. Planning may enable you to set and follow your goals and objectives and build a vision, a strategy, and a routine for your future. Here are some of the benefits of celebrating and planning for your health and mind:

Body: Celebrating and planning can help you to improve your physical health and appearance, as they can help you to maintain and maximize your food, exercise, and lifestyle habits, and prevent or reverse any health issues or hazards. Celebrating and preparing can also help you to improve your body image and self-esteem, as they can help you to recognize and embrace your strengths and beauty, and overcome any insecurities or obstacles.

Mind: Celebrating and planning can help you to improve your mental health and performance, as they can aid you to reduce stress and inflammation, and boost mood and sleep quality. Celebrating and planning can also help you to increase your cognitive function and memory since they can help you stimulate and challenge your brain and learn new skills and knowledge.

As you can see, celebrating and planning can have beneficial consequences on your health and well-being, and your body and mind. To reap these rewards, you need to celebrate your achievements plan for the future, and enjoy the process and the outcome.

How to Celebrate and Plan?

On Day 7, you should focus on celebrating your achievements and planning for the future, and enjoy the process and the outcome. You should also assess the accomplishments and results that you have made in the past week, and congratulate yourself for taking action and making great changes in your life. You should also find out what strategies and suggestions you can use to maintain and enhance your gut health and weight reduction in the long term, such as keeping a food diary, making reasonable goals, tracking your measurements, and rewarding yourself.

Here are some stages that you can follow or adjust according to your preferences and availability:

- **Review:** Review the progress and accomplishments that you have made in the past week, and compare them with your baseline and expectations. You can utilize numerous strategies to measure and evaluate your progress and results, such as:

- **Food diary:** A food diary is a record of what you eat and drink each day, and how you feel before and after. A food journal can assist you in monitoring and analyzing your diet, and spot any patterns, trends, or changes. You can use a food diary app or notepad to record your entries, and then examine them at the end of the week.

- **Goals:** Goals are specific, quantifiable, achievable, relevant, and time-bound statements that outline what you want to do and why. Goals can enable you to focus and direct your actions and track and assess your outcomes. You can use a goal-setting tool or spreadsheet to create and update your goals, and then review them at the end of the week.

- **Measurements:** Measurements are the numerical or qualitative indications that reveal your physical or mental status or change. Measurements can assist you in quantifying and comparing your outcomes, and see your improvement or decline. You can use a measuring tape, a scale, a caliper, or a tracker to take and record your measurements, such as your weight, waist circumference, body fat percentage, or blood pressure, and examine them at the end of the week.

- **Celebrate:** Celebrate the progress and results that you have accomplished in the past week, and praise yourself for taking action and making great changes in your life.

You can utilize numerous techniques to celebrate and congratulate oneself, such as:

- **Compliment:** A compliment is a nice and sincere statement that appreciates or admires someone or something. A complement can allow you to acknowledge and appreciate your work and achievements, and enhance your confidence, motivation, and happiness. You can complement yourself each day, such as "I am proud of myself for eating healthy and exercising regularly", or "I am happy with myself for losing weight.

- **Reward:** A reward is a pleasant and desirable thing or experience that is given or received in return for anything done or attained. A reward can help you reinforce and support your excellent behaviors and accomplishments and make you feel satisfied and fulfilled. You can give yourself a treat each week, such as a new book, a movie, a massage, or a trip, and enjoy it without guilt or regret.

- **Plan:** Plan for the future and build a vision, a strategy, and a routine for your long-term gut health and weight loss, and your general health and well-being. You can use different tools and approaches to plan for the future, such as:

- **Vision board:** A vision board is a collage of images, words, and symbols that reflect your goals and dreams, and encourage you to achieve them. A vision board may allow you to see and manifest your preferred future, and drive you to take action and make it happen. You can make a vision board using a poster, a cork board, or a digital device, and display it in a prominent and accessible spot, such as your bedroom, your office, or your phone.

- **Strategy:** A strategy is a plan of action or way of reaching a goal or solving a problem. A plan can allow you to organize and prioritize your actions, and overcome any hurdles or challenges. You can build a strategy using a spreadsheet, a calendar, or a planner, and update it regularly, such as weekly, monthly, or quarterly.

- **Routine:** A routine is a regular and fixed way of doing anything, such as eating, exercising, or sleeping. A routine can allow you to form and maintain your habits, and generate consistency and stability in your life. You can build a routine using a checklist, a timer, or a reminder, and follow it regularly, such as morning, afternoon, or evening.

On Day 7, you should also enjoy a sample menu for the day that contains your favorite foods from the previous days, and allow yourself some indulgences in moderation. You should also practice some restorative exercises such as stretching, foam rolling, and meditation to heal and revitalize.

Here is a sample menu for the day that you can follow or adapt according to your preferences and availability:

- **Breakfast:** A smoothie bowl made with banana, almond milk, vanilla protein powder, and chia seeds, topped with blueberries, granola, and coconut flakes, followed by a cup of green tea with some honey and lemon.

- **Snack:** A piece of dark chocolate and a cup of coffee with some milk and stevia.

- **Lunch:** A turkey and cheese sandwich made with whole wheat bread, turkey, cheese, lettuce, tomato, and mustard, served with some baby carrots and hummus.

- **Snack:** A handful of mixed nuts and dried fruits, and a cup of herbal tea with a spoonful of honey. This snack can assist you in fulfilling your sweet taste and supply you with some healthy fats, protein, and antioxidants. Nuts and dried fruits are rich in fiber, omega-3 fatty acids, and vitamin E, which can aid your digestion, inflammation, and skin health. Herbal tea and honey are calming and anti-inflammatory, which can assist you to relax and reduce tension. Enjoy this snack and feel the advantages of these super foods and antioxidants.

You have done a terrific job in the previous week, and you should celebrate your achievements and plan for the future. You have learned how to improve your gut health and weight reduction by following a balanced and nutritious diet and engaging in some physical and mental workouts. You have also learned how to reduce stress and inflammation and boost your healing process and protection from free radicals and oxidative damage. You have made excellent adjustments in your life, and you should be pleased with yourself.

To maintain and improve your gut health and weight reduction in the long run, you should continue to practice what you have learned in the previous week, and make it a part of your lifestyle.

Here are some recommendations and advice that can help you to do that:

- **Keep a food journal:** Keeping a food diary can allow you to document what you eat and drink, and how it affects your gut health and weight reduction. You can use a food diary app or notepad to record your meals, snacks, and beverages, and jot down your portions, calories, nutrients, and ingredients. You can also write down how you feel after eating or drinking, such as your energy, mood, digestion, and cravings. This can enable you to discover and adjust your eating habits and patterns and avoid foods that can trigger or worsen your digestive difficulties and weight gain.

- **Set reasonable objectives:** Setting realistic goals might help you to stay motivated and focused on your gut health and weight loss quest. You can use goal-setting software or a notebook to jot down your short-term and long-term goals and break them down into precise, measurable, attainable, relevant, and time-bound (SMART) steps. You may also track your progress and outcomes, and alter your goals and techniques as appropriate. You should also celebrate your achievements and reward yourself for your efforts, such as purchasing yourself a new wardrobe, going for a spa day, or taking a vacation.

- **Track your measurements:** Tracking your measurements can allow you to track your gut health and weight reduction, and see the changes in your body and health. You can use a measuring tape, a scale, a body fat analyzer, or a fitness tracker to measure your waist circumference, weight, body fat percentage, and other markers of your gut health and weight reduction. You can also snap images of yourself before and after your 7-day journey, and compare them to observe the difference. You should also pay attention to how you feel, such as your energy, mood, digestion, and immunity, and how they improve with time.

- **Reward yourself:** Rewarding yourself can enable you to enjoy your gut health and weight reduction journey, and minimize boredom and burnout. You can treat yourself to some indulgences in moderation, such as your favorite meals, drinks, or hobbies, as long as they do not threaten your gut health and weight loss. You can also try new foods, drinks, or activities, that can increase your gut health and weight loss, such as super foods, antioxidants, or fun exercises. You should also have fun and socialize with your friends and family, and share your experiences and achievements with them.

By following these ideas and recommendations, you may maintain and enhance your gut health and weight reduction in the long run, and experience a trimmer tummy, a happier stomach, and a healthier you.

To celebrate your achievements and prepare for the future, you should also enjoy a tasty and nutritious menu for the day, that incorporates your favorite foods from the previous days, and gives you some indulgences in moderation. **Here is a sample menu for the day that you can follow or adapt according to your preferences and availability:**

- **Breakfast:** A smoothie bowl made with avocado, spinach, almond milk, vanilla protein powder, and honey, topped with blueberries, walnuts, and chia seeds, followed by a cup of green tea with some honey and lemon.

- **Snack:** A piece of dark chocolate and a cup of coffee with some coconut oil and stevia.

- **Lunch:** A chicken and veggie wrap made with whole wheat tortilla, hummus, lettuce, tomato, cucumber, olives, feta cheese, and chicken, served with some baked sweet potato fries and ketchup.

- **Snack:** A handful of goji berries and a cup of ginger tea with a slice of lemon.

- **Dinner:** A pizza cooked with whole wheat dough, tomato sauce, mozzarella cheese, mushrooms, spinach, and turkey pepperoni, served with some green salad with some olive oil and vinegar.

- **Snack:** A cup of warm milk with a touch of cinnamon and nutmeg, and a piece of dark chocolate. You can add some lemon, cucumber, mint, or berries to your water to make it more refreshing and delectable.

To celebrate your achievements and prepare for the future, you should also engage in certain restorative activities that can help to heal and rejuvenate your body and mind, which are important for your weight loss and well-being. You should also avoid excessive or vigorous exercises that can create stress or injury to your body.

Stretching: Stretching is a moderate and soothing exercise that can assist in improving your flexibility, mobility, and posture, and reduce stress and inflammation. Stretching can also assist in enhancing your mood and sleep quality since it can produce endorphins and serotonin, which are the hormones that can make you feel joyful and relaxed. You can stretch for at least 10 minutes a day, preferably in the morning or evening, and in a big and pleasant environment. You can utilize your own body weight or add some props, such as a mat, a strap, or a foam roller, to improve the range of motion and challenge. You can follow a stretching video or app, or join a stretching class or group.

Foam rolling: Foam rolling is a self-massage technique that can assist in easing pain and stiffness, and enhance your blood flow and lymphatic drainage. Foam rolling can also help to reduce stress and inflammation, as it can lower your cortisol and cytokine levels, and boost your endorphin and oxytocin levels, which are the hormones that can make you feel relaxed, joyful, and connected. You can foam roll for at least 10 minutes a day, particularly in the evening or before bed, and in a pleasant and peaceful location. You can use a foam roller or a ball, to deliver pressure and movement to your muscles and joints. You can also use some oil, lotion, or cream, to lubricate and nourish your skin.

Meditation: Meditation is the discipline of focusing your attention on a single object, such as your breath, a word, a sound, or a sensation, and observing your thoughts and feelings without judgment or reaction. Meditation can help you reduce stress and inflammation since it can lower your cortisol and cytokine levels, and boost your endorphin and oxytocin levels, which are the hormones that can make you feel calm, joyful, and connected. Meditation can also help you to enhance your mood and sleep quality, as it can increase your serotonin and melatonin levels, which are the hormones that can regulate your mood and sleep cycle. Meditation can also help you to improve your digestion, immunity, and metabolism since it can strengthen your parasympathetic nervous system, which is the rest-and-digest response. To practice meditation, you can sit or lie down in a comfortable and quiet spot, focus on your breath, a word, a sound, or a sensation, and let go of any distractions or judgments. You can meditate for at least 10 minutes a day, preferably in the morning or evening, and utilize a meditation app or video to guide you. These are some of the exercises that you can conduct on Day 7 to celebrate your achievements and plan for the future. However, you should also listen to your body and adapt your intensity and length according to your level and condition. You should also rest and sleep well, as sleep is vital for your body's repair and renewal.

Congratulations! You have completed your 7-day journey to a trimmer tummy, a happy gut, and a healthier you! You have learned how to improve your gut health and weight reduction by following a balanced and nutritious diet and engaging in some physical and mental workouts. You have also learned how to reduce stress and inflammation and boost your healing process and protection from free radicals and oxidative damage. You have made excellent adjustments in your life, and you should be pleased with yourself. You have achieved a trimmer tummy, a happy gut, and a healthier you!

We hope you liked this experience and found it helpful and enlightening. We also hope you will continue to apply what you have learned in the previous week and make it a part of your lifestyle. Remember, you are strong and capable, and you deserve to be well and happy. **Thank you!**

www.ingramcontent.com/pod-product-compliance
Lightning Source LLC
Chambersburg PA
CBHW070854260726
48661CB00004B/1398